Obstetrics/ Gynecology
Nutrition Handbook

Obstetrics/ Gynecology
Nutrition Handbook

Deborah Pesicka, RD, CDE

Judith Riley, MD

Cynthia Thomson, MS, RD, CNSD

Chapman & Hall Nutrition Handbooks 1

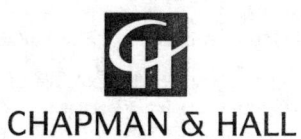

CHAPMAN & HALL

New York • Albany • Bonn • Boston • Cincinnati • Detroit • London • Madrid • Melbourne
Mexico City • Pacific Grove • Paris • San Francisco • Singapore • Tokyo • Toronto • Washington

Cover Design: Andrea Meyer, emDASH inc.

Copyright © 1996
Chapman & Hall

Printed in the United States of America

For more information, contact:

Chapman & Hall
115 Fifth Avenue
New York, NY 10003

Chapman & Hall
2-6 Boundary Row
London SE1 8HN
England

1 2 3 4 5 6 7 8 9 10 XXX 01 00 99 97 96 95

Library of Congress Cataloging-in-Publication Data

Pesicka, Deborah, 1956-
    Obstetrics/gynecology nutrition handbook / Deborah Pesicka, Judith Riley, and Cynthia Thomson
        p.   cm. — (Chapman & Hall nutrition handbooks : 1)
    Includes bibliographical references.
    ISBN 0–412–07501–6
    1. Pregnancy—Nutrition aspects—Handbooks, manuals, etc.
2. Puerperium—Nutritional aspects—Handbooks, manuals, etc.   3. Lactation—Nutritional aspects—Handbooks, manuals, etc.   I. Riley, Judith, 1954-   .
II. Thomson, Cynthia, 1957-   .   III. Title.   IV. Series.
RM217.2.C44   1996 vol. 1
[RG559]
615.8'54   s—dc20
[618.2'4]
DNLM/DLC   95–16241
for Library of Congress   CIP

British Library Cataloguing in Publication Data available

To order for this or any other Chapman & Hall book, please contact **International Thomson Publishing, 7625 Empire Drive, Florence, KY 41042.** Phone: (606) 525-6600. Fax: (606) 525-7778, e-mail: order@chaphall.com.

For a complete listing of Chapman & Hall's titles, send your requests to **Chapman & Hall, Dept. BC, 115 Fifth Avenue, New York, NY 10003.**

Preface

Current knowledge of the role of nutrition in the care of pregnant and lactating women continues to expand. There is now clear evidence that nutrition can directly affect both pregnancy outcome and lactation performance. It is imperative that health care professionals integrate nutrition and assessment of the adequacy of each patient's diet into the routine care of pregnant and lactating women in order to optimize their health and the health of the infant.

This handbook was developed by health care professionals in nutrition and obstetrics/gynecology to provide health care professionals with essential information for the nutritional care of women. This handbook provides the tools for effective evaluation of each patient's nutritional status, initiation of an appropriate nutritional care plan, and monitoring of nutritional care.

We would like to thank Julia Meyer, not only for her data entry assistance, but also for sharing a medical student's perspective in the development of the handbook contents. We would also like to express our gratitude to Kathleen Jaegers for her thoroughness and word processing expertise in the design and development of this handbook.

This handbook was made possible through NIH/NCI Grant No. CA-53459, Nutrition Education Curriculum for the Medical School.

We hope you will find this handbook to be a valuable tool in providing care to your obstetrics patients.

Deborah Pesicka RD, CDE
   Clinical Dietician
University Medical Center
Cynthia Thomson, MS, RD, CNSD
   Program Coordinator, Nutrition Curriculum
in Medical Education
   Department of Family and Community Medicine
   University of Arizona, Tucson

Table of Contents

List of Tables and Figures

Abbreviations

BMI	body mass index
BS	blood sugar
°C	degrees centigrade
cm	centimeter
C-section	Cesarean section
dL	deciliter
°F	degrees Fahrenheit
GDM	Gestational Diabetes Mellitus
G.I.	gastrointestinal
gm	gram
Hct	hematocrit
Hgb	hemoglobin
IBW	ideal body weight
ICU	intensive care unit
IgA	immunoglobulin A
IgG	immunoglobulin G
IgM	immunoglobulin M
IU	international unit
IUP	intrauterine pregnancy
kcal	kilocalorie
kg	kilogram
lb	pound
LBW	low birth weight
MCHC	mean corpuscular hemoglobin concentration
MCV	mean corpuscular volume
mEq	milliequivalent
mg	milligram
ml	milliliter
NAS	National Academy of Sciences
ng	nanogram
ob/gyn	obstetrics/gynecology
oz	ounce
PKU	phenylketonuria
RBC	red blood cell
RDA	Recommended Dietary Allowances
SIADH	Syndrome of Inappropriate Antidiuretic Hormone
svg	serving

Tbsp .... tablespoon
tsp .... teaspoon
μg .... microgram
USDA .... United States Department of Agriculture
WIC .... Women, Infants, and Children
wk .... week
y/o .... years old
yr .... year
⇓ .... decreased
⇑ .... increased

SECTION 1
Nutrition at Prenatal and Postnatal Checkups

Table 1.1
NUTRITIONAL CARE AT PRENATAL AND POSTNATAL CHECKUPS

Visit	Assessment	Counseling/Reference Info
First prenatal visit	• Pregnancy history for low birth weight and premature births	• p. 22, Clinical recommendations • p. 7, Daily Food Guide
6–12 wk IUP	• Measure height and weight	• p. 22, Clinical recommendations • p. 23, Prenatal weight gain chart
	• Plot or calculate BMI	• p. 23, BMI • p. 24, Set weight gain goals with patient
	• Exercise during pregnancy	• p. 35, Exercise
	• Evaluate use of alcohol, tobacco, and drugs	• p. 26, Effects of alcohol, tobacco, and illegal drug use
	• Evaluate caffeine intake	• p. 36, Effects of caffeine
	• Evaluate diet; start prenatal vitamin/mineral supplement	• p. 7, Daily Food Guide • p. 10,11,12, Vitamin/mineral supplementation
	• Plans to breastfeed	• p. 42, Advantages of breastfeeding
12–18 wk	• Evaluate for problems with nausea, emesis, etc.	• p. 34,35, Common complaints during pregnancy
	• Evaluate weight gain	• p. 23,24, BMI, weight assessment • p. 26, Nutrition referral as indicated

Table 1.1

NUTRITIONAL CARE AT PRENATAL AND POSTNATAL CHECKUPS *Continued*

18–24 wk	• Evaluate weight gain
	• Evaluate for anemia
	
	• Evaluate for calcium intake
		• p. 23,24, BMI, weight assessment
		• p. 31, Diagnostic criteria for anemia
		  p. 28, WIC referral if indicated
		  p. 16, Iron sources
		  p. 16, Folate sources
		• p. 14, Calcium sources

24–28 wk	• Evaluate weight gain • Evaluate blood glucose • Evaluate for common problems during pregnancy	• p. 23,24, BMI, weight assessment • p. 38, Diagnostic criteria for GDM p. 26, Nutrition referral as indicated • p. 34,35, Intervention for common problems
29–40 wk	• Repeat measures of weight gain • Plans to breastfeed	• p. 23,24, BMI, weight assessment • p. 42, Advantages to breastfeeding p. 45,46, Diet during lactation
Delivery	• Diet • Plans to exercise	• p. 14, Calcium • p. 15, Fiber • p. 16, Folate • p. 16, Iron • p. 17, Protein • p. 17, Sodium • p. 18,19,20, Vitamins A, B_6, B_{12}, C, and D • p. 20, Zinc • p. 42, Postpartum healing • p. 44, Postpartum exercise

continued on next page

Table 1.1
NUTRITIONAL CARE AT PRENATAL AND POSTNATAL CHECKUPS *Continued*

Visit	Assessment	Counseling/Reference Info
Postpartum	• Weight status	• p. 44, Postpartum exercise
		p. 43, Postpartum weight loss
		p. 43, Nutritious snacks
	• Progress with breastfeeding	• p. 47, Breastfeeding basics
		p. 46, Foods/beverages consumed during lactation which may cause infant G.I. distress
		p. 48, Breastfeeding concerns, tips
		p. 46, Nutrition referral
		p. 51, Breastfeeding resources

SECTION 2
Nutritional Requirements During Pregnancy and Lactation

Food Guide Pyramid and Daily Food Guide

Food Guide Pyramid

The Food Guide Pyramid was developed by the United States Department of Agriculture (USDA) in 1992 to provide Americans with a visual tool for healthy eating. The Pyramid (Figure 2.1) is based on scientific research of what Americans eat, what nutrients are in various foods, and how to make the best food choices for optimal health.

Figure 2.1

Food Guide Pyramid

The **Food Guide Pyramid** emphasizes foods from the five food groups shown in the three lower sections of the Pyramid.

Each of these food groups provides some, but not all, of the nutrients you need. Foods in one group can't replace those in another. No one food group is more important than another—for good health, you need them all.

A Guide to Daily Food Choices

The Pyramid is an outline of what to eat each day. It's not a rigid prescription, but a general guide that lets you choose a healthful diet that's right for you. The Pyramid calls for eating a variety of foods to get the nutrients you need and at the same time the right amount of calories to maintain a healthy weight.

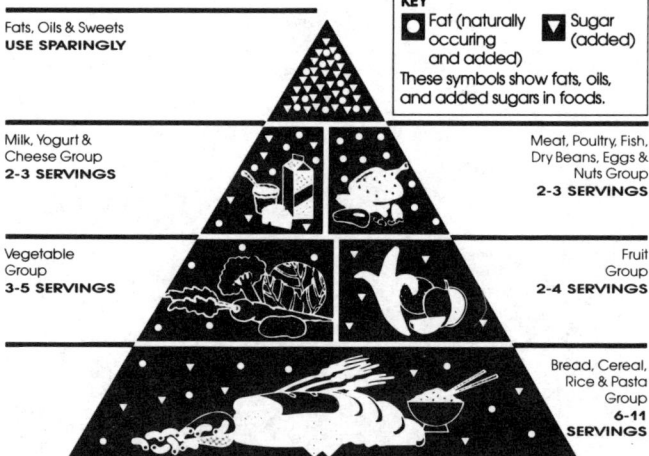

KEY
◻ Fat (naturally occuring and added)   ▼ Sugar (added)
These symbols show fats, oils, and added sugars in foods.

Fats, Oils & Sweets
USE SPARINGLY

Milk, Yogurt & Cheese Group
2-3 SERVINGS

Meat, Poultry, Fish, Dry Beans, Eggs & Nuts Group
2-3 SERVINGS

Vegetable Group
3-5 SERVINGS

Fruit Group
2-4 SERVINGS

Bread, Cereal, Rice & Pasta Group
6-11 SERVINGS

Source: U.S. Department of Agriculture and the U.S. Department of Health and Human Resources, Food Guide Pyramid: A Guide to Daily Food Choices, National Live Stock and Meat Board, Washington, DC. Copyright © 1993.

Daily Food Guide

The Daily Food Guide provides guidelines for the number of servings from each food group which should be eaten daily during pregnancy and lactation.

		Number of Servings		
Food Group	Serving Size	During Adolescent Pregnancy	During Pregnancy	During Lactation
Breads/ Cereals/ Rice/ Pasta	1/2 cup cooked rice, cereal, or pasta; 1 slice bread; 4 crackers	9–11	6–11	6–11
Fats/ Oils/ Sweets	1 tsp margarine, mayonnaise, salad dressing, or gravy	use in moderation	use sparingly	use sparingly
Fruits	1 small piece fresh fruit; 1/2 cup canned fruit; 1/3 cup fruit juice	2–4	2–4	2–4
Milk/ Dairy	1 cup milk, cottage cheese, or yogurt; 1 oz cheese	5	4	4
Protein-rich	3 oz meat, fish, or poultry; 1 cup dried beans	4	3–4	3–4
Vege-tables	1/2 cup fresh, cooked, or canned	3–5	3–5	3–5

Table 2.1
DAILY FOOD GUIDE

Recommended Dietary Allowances

"Recommended Dietary Allowances (RDA) are the levels of intake of essential nutrients considered in the judgment of the Committee on Dietary Allowances of the Food and Nutrition Board, on the basis of available scientific knowledge, to be adequate to meet or exceed known nutritional needs of practically all *healthy persons*."

RDAs (see Table 2.2) reflect the average daily intakes which populations should consume over time and are not individual requirements.

Micronutrient and Mineral Requirements

Table 2.3 indicates the nutrients for which the RDA is increased during pregnancy and/or lactation. Note that pregnant adolescents have increased nutrient requirements related to both their own growth and the growth of the fetus.

Energy Requirements

During Pregnancy: The current RDA for energy during pregnancy is for an additional 300 kcal/day beginning at the second trimester of pregnancy. The daily energy requirements of pregnancy increase throughout pregnancy related to increased fetal size, increased maternal energy expenditure, and increased maternal fat stores. Pregnant women may meet energy requirements by increasing caloric consumption, by reducing activity, or through a combination of increasing caloric intake and reducing energy expenditure.

During Lactation: Energy requirements during lactation are estimated to be 850 kcal/day to produce an adequate breast milk supply for the growing infant: 500 kcal should be consumed as nutrient dense foods (i.e., foods which provide the additional calcium, protein, and B vitamins needed during lactation), and the remaining 350 kcal may be derived from maternal fat stores accumulated during pregnancy.

Table 2.2
RECOMMENDED DIETARY ALLOWANCES^a

Category	Age (yrs)	Weight^b (kg)	(lb)	Height^b (cm)	(in)	Protein (gm)	Vitamin A (μg RE)^c	Vitamin D (μg)^d	Vitamin E (mg α-TE)^e	Vitamin K (μg)
Infants	0.0–0.5	6	13	60	24	13	375	7.5	3	5
	0.5–1.0	9	20	71	28	14	375	10	4	10
Children	1–3	13	29	90	35	16	400	10	6	15
	4–6	20	44	112	44	24	500	10	7	20
	7–10	28	62	132	52	28	700	10	7	30
Males	11–14	45	99	157	62	45	1,000	10	10	45
	15–18	66	145	176	69	59	1,000	10	10	65
	19–24	72	160	177	70	58	1,000	10	10	70
	25–50	79	174	176	70	63	1,000	5	10	80
	51+	77	170	173	68	63	1,000	5	10	80
Females	11–14	46	101	157	62	46	800	10	8	45
	15–18	55	120	163	64	44	800	10	8	55
	19–24	58	128	164	65	46	800	10	8	60
	25–50	63	138	163	64	50	800	5	8	65
	51+	65	143	160	63	50	800	5	8	65
Pregnant						60	800	10	10	65
Lactating										
1st 6 months						65	1,300	10	12	65
2nd 6 months						62	1,200	10	11	65

continued on next page

Table 2.2
RECOMMENDED DIETARY ALLOWANCES[a] Continued

Category	Age (yrs)	Weight (kg)	Weight (lb)	Height (cm)	Height (in)	Protein (gm)	Vitamin C (mg)	Thiamine (mg)	Riboflavin (mg)	Niacin (mg NE)	Vitamin B₆ (mg)	Folate (µg)	Vitamin B₁₂ (µg)
Infants	0.0–0.5	6	13	60	24	13	30	0.3	0.4	5	0.3	25	0.3
	0.5–1.0	9	20	71	28	14	35	0.4	0.5	6	0.6	35	0.5
Children	1–3	13	29	90	35	16	40	0.7	0.8	9	1.0	50	0.7
	4–6	20	44	112	44	24	45	0.9	1.1	12	1.1	75	1.0
	7–10	28	62	132	52	28	45	1.0	1.2	13	1.4	100	1.4
Males	11–14	45	99	157	62	45	50	1.3	1.5	17	1.7	150	2.0
	15–18	66	145	176	69	59	60	1.5	1.8	20	2.0	200	2.0
	19–24	72	160	177	70	58	60	1.5	1.7	19	2.0	200	2.0
	25–50	79	174	176	70	63	60	1.5	1.7	19	2.0	200	2.0
	51+	77	170	173	68	63	60	1.2	1.4	15	2.0	200	2.0
Females	11–14	46	101	157	62	46	50	1.1	1.3	15	1.4	150	2.0
	15–18	55	120	163	64	44	60	1.1	1.3	15	1.5	180	2.0
	19–24	58	128	164	65	46	60	1.1	1.3	15	1.6	180	2.0
	25–50	63	138	163	64	50	60	1.1	1.3	15	1.6	180	2.0
	51+	65	143	160	63	50	70	1.0	1.2	13	1.6	180	2.0
Pregnant						60	70	1.5	1.6	17	2.2	400	2.2
Lactating 1st 6 months						65	95	1.6	1.8	20	2.1	280	2.6
2nd 6 months						62	90	1.6	1.7	20	2.1	260	2.6

Table 2.2
RECOMMENDED DIETARY ALLOWANCES *Continued*

^{a}The allowances, expressed as average daily intakes over time, are intended to provide for individual variations among most normal persons as they live in the United States under usual environmental stresses. Diets should be based on a variety of common foods in order to provide other nutrients for which human requirements have been less well defined.

^{b}Weights and heights of Reference Adults are actual medians for the US population of the designated age, as reported by NHANES II. The use of these figures does not imply that the height-to-weight ratios are ideal.

^{c}Retinol equivalents. 1 retinol equivalent = 1 μg retinol or 6 μg β-carotene.

^{d}As cholecalciferol. 10 μg cholecalciferol = 400 IU of vitamin D.

^{e}α-Tocopherol equivalents. 1 mg d-α tocopherol = 1α-TE.

^{f}1 NE (biacin equivalent) is equal to 1 mg of niacin or 60 mg of dietary tryptophan.

SUMMARY TABLE Estimated Safe and Adequate Daily Dietary Intakes of Selected Vitamins and Minerals^a

		Vitamins		Trace Elements^b				
Category	Age (yrs)	Biotin (μg)	Pantothenic Acid (mg)	Copper (mg)	Manganese (mg)	Fluoride (mg)	Chromium (μg)	Molybdenum (μg)
Infants	0–0.5	10	2	0.4–0.6	0.3–0.6	0.1–0.5	10–40	15–30
	0.5–1	15	3	0.6–0.7	0.6–1.0	0.2–1.0	20–60	20–40
Children and adolescents	1–3	20	3	0.7–1.0	1.0–1.5	0.5–1.5	20–80	25–50
	4–6	25	3–4	1.0–1.5	1.5–2.0	1.0–2.5	30–120	30–75
	7–10	30	4–5	1.0–2.0	2.0–3.0	1.5–2.5	50–200	50–150
	11+	30–100	4–7	1.5–2.5	2.0–5.0	1.5–2.5	50–200	75–250
Adults		30–100	4–7	1.5–3.0	2.0–5.0	1.5–4.0	50–200	75–250

^{a}Because there is less information on which to base allowances, these figures are not given in the main table of RDA and are provided here in the form of ranges of recommended intakes.

^{b}Since the toxic levels for many trace elements may be only several times usual intakes, the upper levels for the trace elements given in this table should not be habitually exceeded.

Reprinted with permission from Recommended Dietary Allowances: 10th ed. Copyright 1989 by the National Academy of Sciences. Courtesy of the National Academy Press, Washington, DC.

Table 2.2
RECOMMENDED DIETARY ALLOWANCES[a] Continued

		Weight[b]		Height[b]					Minerals				
Category	Age (yrs)	(kg)	(lb)	(cm)	(in)	Pro-tein (gm)	Cal-cium (mg)	Phos-phorus (mg)	Mag-nesium (mg)	Iron (mg)	Zinc (mg)	Iodine (µg)	Sele-nium (µg)
Infants	0.0–0.5	6	13	60	24	13	400	300	40	6	5	40	10
	0.5–1.0	9	20	71	28	14	600	500	60	10	5	50	15
Children	1–3	13	29	90	35	16	800	800	80	10	10	70	20
	4–6	20	44	112	44	24	800	800	120	10	10	90	20
	7–10	28	62	132	52	28	800	800	170	10	10	120	30
Males	11–14	45	99	157	62	45	1,200	1,200	270	12	15	150	40
	15–18	66	145	176	69	59	1,200	1,200	400	12	15	150	50
	19–24	72	160	177	70	58	1,200	1,200	350	10	15	150	70
	25–50	79	174	176	70	63	800	800	350	10	15	150	70
	51+	77	170	173	68	63	800	800	350	10	15	150	70
Females	11–14	46	101	157	62	46	1,200	1,200	280	15	12	150	45
	15–18	55	120	163	64	44	1,200	1,200	300	15	12	150	50
	19–24	58	128	164	65	46	1,200	1,200	280	15	12	150	55
	25–50	63	138	163	64	50	800	800	280	15	12	150	55
	51+	65	143	160	63	50	800	800	280	10	12	150	55
Pregnant						60	1,200	1,200	320	30	15	175	65
Lactating													
1st 6 months						65	1,200	1,200	355	15	19	200	75
2nd 6 months						62	1,200	1,200	340	15	16	200	75

continued on next page

Table 2.3
VITAMIN AND MINERAL REQUIREMENTS DURING PREGNANCY

	Adolescent Pregnancy	Pregnancy	Lactation	Recommendations for Daily Intake
VITAMINS				
Folate	400 µg	400 µg	280 µg	Whole grains, dried beans, green vegetables, organ meats—daily
Vitamin A	800 mg	800 mg	1300 mg	Yellow or orange fruits and vegetables—at least once/day
Vitamin B_6	2.2 mg	2.1 mg	2.1 mg	Whole grains, dried beans, dark greens, meats—liberally
Vitamin C	70 mg	70 mg	95 mg	Citrus fruits, strawberries, cantaloupe, tomatoes, potatoes at least once/day
Vitamin D	15 µg	10 µg	10 µg	Milk or milk products at least 4 svgs/day; exposure to sunlight
MINERALS				
Calcium	1600 mg	1200 mg	1200 mg	Low-fat/non-fat milk and milk products; greens, sardines, salmon w/bones—at least 4 svgs/day. Adolescent pregnancy—5 svgs/day
Iron	30 mg	30 mg	15 mg	Organ meats, red meats, fish, poultry, fortified cereals, enriched breads, spinach 2-4 svgs/day; supplement as indicated
Zinc	19 mg	15 mg	19 mg	Red meats, seafood, oysters—daily

Source: Recommend Dietary Allowances (for intake levels)

13

Protein Requirements

During Pregnancy: The RDA for protein during pregnancy is an additional 10 gm/day during the second and third trimesters. This increased requirement can be met by consuming daily an additional 10 oz of low-fat milk, or an additional 1.5 oz of lean meat or low-fat cheese.

During Lactation: The lactating mother should consume an additional 15 gm of protein daily to meet the protein requirements related to breast milk production. This increased requirement can be met by consuming daily 16 oz of low-fat milk, 2 oz of lean meat, 2oz of low-fat cheese, 1/2 cup of cottage cheese, or 1 cup of cooked beans.

Vitamin and Mineral Supplementation

The National Academy of Sciences' (NAS) publication, *Nutrition During Pregnancy and Lactation: An Implementation Guide*, indicates that routine assessment of dietary practices is recommended for all pregnant women in the United States. Prenatal vitamin and mineral supplements are indicated for high risk populations and for pregnant women with inadequate diets. The NAS' report recommends that these individuals receive a dailymultivitamin/mineral supplement containing the nutrients listed in Table 2.4, beginning in the second trimester.

Supplements containing high levels of folate or iron negatively affect zinc metabolism during pregnancy; therefore, prenatal vitamins should contain adequate levels of zinc. Women receiving supplemental iron (>30 mg/day) should also receive supplemental zinc (15mg/day) and copper (2 mg/day).

Table 2.4 NAS' VITAMIN/MINERAL SUPPLEMENT RECOMMENDATIONS			
Calcium	250 mg	Vitamin B_6	2 mg
Copper	2 mg	Vitamin C	50 mg
Folate	300 µg	Vitamin D	10 µg
Iron	30–60 mg	Zinc	15 mg

Adapted with permission from Institute of Medicine. Nutrition During Pregnancy and Lactation: An Implementation Guide, *National Academy Press: Washington, DC, 1992.*

Table 2.5 PRENATAL VITAMIN/MINERAL NUTRIENT ANALYSIS (MATERNA®*)			
Biotin	30 µg	Pantothenic acid	10 mg
Calcium (carbonate)	250 mg	Pyridoxine	10 mg
Chromium	25 µg	Riboflavin	3.4 mg
Copper	2 mg	Thiamin	3 mg
Folate	1 mg	Vitamin A	5000 IU
Iodine	150 µg	Vitamin B_{12}	20 µg
Iron	60 mg	Vitamin C	100 mg
Magnesium	25 mg	Vitamin D	400 IU
Manganese	5 mg	Vitamin E	30 IU
Molybdenum	25 µg	Zinc	25 mg
Niacin	20 mg		

*Data from product label.

Case reports have suggested an association between high doses of vitamin A ($\geq$25,000 IU) during pregnancy and birth defects. Supplementation with 8000 IU vitamin A should be considered the maximum intake prior to or during pregnancy.

Many obstetricians routinely prescribe prenatal vitamin/mineral supplementation to pregnant and lactating women (1 tablet daily) to promote adequate micronutrient intake. Table 2.5 lists the nutrient composition of one such prenatal vitamin/mineral supplement (Materna®). Many patients will also have inadequate iron intake. Dietary iron intake should be assessed (see Table 3.5) and anemia evaluation completed as indicated (see Table 5.2).

Vitamin and Mineral Supplements

The use of nutritional supplements depends on a variety of factors including the presence of anemia, the age of the mother, diet history, family history of neural tube defects, smoking, multiple gestation, vegetarianism, and so forth. Table 2.6 describes these factors and the recommended nutrient supplementation related to each.

Table 2.6
INDICATIONS FOR NUTRIENT SUPPLEMENTATION

Reproductive Period and Conditions	Iron[a, b] 30 mg (low dose)	Iron[b, c] 60–120 mg	Multivitamin/ Mineral (low dose)	Calcium 600 mg
PRECONCEPTION, INTERCONCEPTION				
Iron deficiency anemia		√	√	
PREGNANCY				
Normal	√		√	
Multiple gestation			√	
Poor quality diet, resistant to change			√	√
Complete vegetarian			√	
Iron-deficiency anemia		√	√	
Alcohol abuse			√	
Heavy cigarette smoking			√	
<25 y/o, consuming no calcium-rich milk products, resistant to change			√[d]	√

Table 2.6
INDICATIONS FOR NUTRIENT SUPPLEMENTATION *Continued*

Reproductive Period and Conditions	Iron[a, b] 30 mg (low dose)	Iron[b, c] 60–120 mg	Multivitamin/ Mineral (low dose)	Calcium 600 mg
LACTATION				
Low intake of energy			√	
Low intake of milk products			√[d]	√
Iron deficiency anemia		√	√	

[a]Begin routine iron supplementation for all pregnant women by the 12th week of gestation.

[b]Iron should be taken with juice or water, apart from meals.

[c]Therapeutic doses of iron should be taken apart from other supplements.

[d]The vitamin supplement is indicated to supply vitamin D. Regular exposure to sunshine reduces the need for this supplement.

Adapted with permission from *Institute of Medicine.* Nutrition During Pregnancy and Lactation: An Implementation Guide. *National Academy Press: Washington, DC, 1992.*

SECTION 3
Food Sources
of Nutrients

Many patients may ask questions as to the best food sources for specific nutrients they may be trying to increase or restrict the intake of. Below and on the following pages of this section are tables to assist in educating patients as to the dietary sources of several key nutrients.

Table 3.1 DIETARY SOURCES OF CALCIUM	
Good: >200 mg	
Food Item	*Svg Size*
Broccoli/Greens*	2 cups
Canned salmon w/bones	3 oz
Canned sardines w/bones*	3 oz
Cheese (cheddar, edam, Monterey jack, mozzarella, Parmesan, provolone, ricotta, Romano, Swiss)	1 oz
Ice cream	1 cup
Ice milk	1 cup
Milk (skim, 2%, whole, buttermilk)	1 cup
Yogurt	6–8 oz
Fair 100–200 mg	
Food Item	*Svg Size*
Almonds	2 oz
Corn muffin	1
Cottage cheese	1 cup
Greens, collard, mustard	1/2 cup
Orange juice (calcium-fortified)	3/4 cup
Other cheeses	1 oz
Sardines	1–2 fish
Spinach	1/2 cup
Tortilla (lime-processed corn or flour)	1 (10 in. diameter)

Generally not as well absorbed.

Table 3.2
DIETARY SOURCES OF FIBER*

Food Item	Svg Size	gm/Svg
Cereals		
All Bran®	1/3 cup	8.8
Bran Buds®	1/3 cup	7.9
Bran cereal	1/2 cup	8.0–13.0
Bran Chex®	2/3 cup	4.6
Cracklin' Bran®	1/2 cup	4.3
Fiber One®	1/3 cup	11.0
Oat bran	1/3 cup	4.0
Raisin bran	3/4 cup	4.0–4.8
Fruits		
Apple	1 medium	3.5
Pear	1 medium	4.1
Raspberries	1/2 cup	2.9
Strawberries	1 cup	3.0
Vegetables		
Avocado	1 medium	4.6
Baked beans	1/2 cup	8.8
Black beans	1/2 cup	4.0
Broccoli	1/2 cup	5.5
Carrots	1 cup	3.1
Green peas	1/2 cup	7.3
Kidney beans	1/2 cup	4.5
Lima beans (cooked)	1/2 cup	2.1
Pinto beans	1/2 cup	3.6
Spinach	1/2 cup	2.1
Zucchini	1/2 cup	1.8
Other		
Popcorn	3 cups	3.0
Whole wheat pasta	1 cup	3.9

*Recommended fiber intake: 25–35 g/day.

Table 3.3
DIETARY SOURCES HIGH IN SOLUBLE AND INSOLUBLE FIBER

Soluble

Apples	Oats and oat bran
Barley	Strawberries
Citrus fruits	

Insoluble

Fresh fruit	Root vegetables
Legumes	Seeds
Nuts	Wheat bran
Raw vegetables	Whole grain breads and cereals

Table 3.4
DIETARY SOURCES OF FOLATE

Excellent: >100 mcg

Food Item	Svg Size
Asparagus	1/2 cup
Baked beans	1 cup
Black-eyed peas	1 cup
Kidney beans	1 cup
Lentils	1 cup
Liver and other organ meats:	
beef	3.5 oz
chicken	3.5 oz
Orange juice	1 cup
Peanuts	4 oz
Spinach	1/2 cup

Good: 15–99 mcg

Food Item	Svg Size
Almonds	4 oz
Beets	1/2 cup
Cantaloupe/Honeydew melon	1 cup
Cauliflower	1/2 cup
Egg	1
Lettuce (romaine)	1/2 cup
Ready-to-eat, fortified cereals	3/4 cup
Turnip greens	1/2 cup
Whole wheat bread	1 slice

Table 3.5
DIETARY SOURCES OF IRON

Excellent: >4 mg

Food Item	Svg Size
Beef liver	3 oz
Clams	1/2 cup
Figs (dried)	10
Iron-fortified cereal	1/2 cup
Iron-fortified infant cereal	3 Tsp
Kidney beans	1 cup
Molasses (blackstrap)	3 Tbsp
Peaches (dried)	10 halves
Pinto beans	1 cup
Ready-to-eat, fortified cereals (like Product 19®, Total®)	3/4 cup
Sunflower seeds (dried, hulled)	2/3 cup

Good: 2–4 mg

Food Item	Svg Size
Beef	3 oz
Egg yolks	3
Iron-fortified infant formula	4 oz
Lamb	3 oz
Lima beans	1/2 cup
Oysters	3 oz
Peas	1 cup
Pork	3 oz
Prune juice	1 cup
Raisins	2/3 cup
Soybeans	1/2 cup

Table 3.6
DIETARY SOURCES OF PROTEIN

Excellent: >20 gm

Food Item	Svg Size	gm/Svg
Chicken (no skin)	3 oz	28
Cod (broiled)	3 oz	23
Cottage cheese	1 cup	26
Hamburger (regular)	3 oz	21
Lamb (roast)	3 oz	23
Pork chop (lean)	3 oz	25
Roast beef	3 oz	25
Shrimp	3 oz	21
Steak (lean)	3 oz	24
Tuna	3 oz	24

Good: 4–18 gms

Food Item	Svg Size	gm/Svg
Beans (dried, cooked)	1 cup	15
Cheeses (low-fat)	3 oz	18
Egg (white)	1 medium	6
Ham	3 oz	18
Milk	1 cup	8
Peanuts	1/4 cup	9
Peanut butter	1 Tbsp	4
Sausage	3 oz	17
Yogurt (low-fat)	1 cup	12

Table 3.7
DIETARY SOURCES OF SODIUM

Food Item	Svg Size	mg/Svg
Breads/Grains/Cereals		
Crackers, chips (salted)	10	250
Meats		
Anchovies, sardines	3 oz	325
Bacon	3 slices	303
Ham	3.5 oz	1300
Hot dogs	1 frank	585
Bologna, other luncheon meats	1-oz slice	226
Sausage	1 link	168
Smoked meats, fish	3 oz	649
Milk/Dairy		
Buttermilk	8 oz	257
Cheese	1 oz	200–400
Cottage cheese	4 oz	457
Vegetables		
Olives	10 medium	350
Pickles, pickle relish (kosher dill)	1 oz	323
Sauerkraut	1/2 cup	780
Other		
Garlic salt	1 tsp	1300
Nuts (salted)	4 oz	700
Saladitos (salted prunes)	5	300
Salt	1 tsp	2300
Soups, bouillon (canned or dried)	8 oz	897
Soy sauce	1 oz	768

Table 3.8
DIETARY SOURCES OF VITAMIN A
(per 1/2 cup serving)

Excellent: 3000 IU

Apricots (dried)	Papaya
Beef liver	Pumpkin
Cantaloupe	Spinach/Other dark green
Carrots	leafy vegetables
Mangoes	Squash
Mixed vegetables	

Good: 1000–3000 IU

Apricot nectar	Nectarine
Asparagus	Purple plums
Broccoli	Sweet potatoes
Chili peppers	

Fair: 500–1000 IU

Apricots (fresh)	Prunes/Prune juice
Brussels sprouts	Tomatoes/Tomato juice
Cheddar cheese	Watermelon
Peaches/Peach nectar	

Table 3.9
DIETARY SOURCES OF VITAMIN B$_6$

Avocado	Oatmeal	Tuna
Beans	Peas	Wheat germ
Bran	Pork	Yams
Cereal (fortified)	Salmon (fresh)	Yeast
Milk (dry skim)	Sweet potatoes	

Table 3.10
DIETARY SOURCES OF VITAMIN B_{12}

Excellent: >1.0 mcg	
Food Item	*Svg Size*
Beef (ground)	3.5 oz
Beef (steaks, roasts)	3.5 oz
Carnation Instant Breakfast®	1 cup (mixed)
Eggnog	1 cup
Fish	3.5 oz
Liver	3.5 oz
Milkshake	1 cup
Veal	3.5 oz
Good: 0.25 - 0.90 mcg	
Food Item	*Svg Size*
Chicken	3.5 oz
Egg	1
Ham	3.5 oz
Lunch meats	3.5 oz
Milk (2%)	1 cup
Pork	3.5 oz
Turkey	3.5 oz
Yogurt (low-fat)	1 cup

Table 3.11
DIETARY SOURCES OF VITAMIN C
(per 1/2 cup serving)

Excellent: 60 mg

Broccoli	Mangoes
Brussels sprouts	Oranges/Orange juice
Cabbage	Papaya
Cauliflower	Peppers
Cranberry juice cocktail	Spinach
Grapefruit/Grapefruit juice	Strawberries
Kiwi	Vitamin C-fortified
Kohlrabi	infant juices

Good: 25–40 mg

Asparagus	Pineapple/Pineapple juice
Bean sprouts (raw)	Potato (with skin)
Cantaloupe	Pureed baby fruits
Chard	Tangerine
Green chili	Tomatoes/Tomato juice
Honeydew melon	

Table 3.12
DIETARY SOURCES OF VITAMIN D*
(per 3 oz serving)

Excellent: >100 IU (2.5 µg)

Fortified cereal	Salmon
Herring, kippers	Sardines
Mackerel	Tuna
Milk	

Good: 50–100 IU (2.5 µg)

Egg	Milkshake (fast-food)
Custard	Pudding
Mazola margarine®	

Note: Exposure to sunlight also provides vitamin D.

Table 3.13
DIETARY SOURCES OF ZINC

Excellent: >4 mg

Food Item	Svg Size	mg/Svg
Beef (lean, cooked)	3 oz	5.1
Calves' liver (cooked)	3 oz	5.3
Lamb (lean, cooked)	3 oz	4.0
Oysters, Atlantic	3 oz	63.0
Oysters, Pacific	3 oz	7.6

Good: 0.9–3.4 mg

Food Item	Svg Size	mg/Svg
Black-eyed peas (cooked)	1/2 cup	3.4
Chicken	3 oz	2.4
Crabmeat	1/2 cup	3.4
Green peas (cooked)	1/2 cup	0.9
Lima beans (cooked)	1/2 cup	0.9
Milk (whole)	1 cup	0.9
Pork loin (cooked)	3 oz	2.6
Potato (baked with skin)	1 medium	1.0
Shrimp	1/2 cup	1.4
Tuna (oil-packed, drained)	3 oz	0.9
Whitefish (broiled)	3 oz	0.9
Yogurt (plain)	1 cup	1.1

SECTION 4
Assessment and Maintenance of Nutritional Status

Pregnancy Weight Gain/Loss

Clinical Recommendations
Weight gain is the single-most reliable indicator of pregnancy outcome. Therefore, weight status should be routinely assessed and close attention paid to the pattern of weight change throughout pregnancy (Table 4.1).

Table 4.1 PREGNANCY WEIGHT GAIN GOALS		
Prepregnancy Ideal Body Weight (IBW)	*Prepregnancy Body Mass Index (BMI)*	*Optimal Weight Gain (in lbs)*
90%	<19.8	28–40
100%	19.8–26.0	25–35
120%	26.1–29.0	15–25
135%	>29.0	≈ 15

Adapted with permission from Institute of Medicine. Nutrition During Pregnancy and Lactation: An Implementation Guide, *National Academy Press: Washington, DC, 1990, p.10.*

Prior to conception:
• Use consistent, reliable procedures to accurately measure and record the woman's weight and height without shoes.
• Plot height and weight to determine her prepregnancy BMI (Figure 4.1).

At the first prenatal visit:
• Estimate the woman's gestational age from the onset of her last menstruation.
• Use consistent, reliable procedures to accurately measure and record her weight and height.
• Plot her height and weight to determine her prenatal BMI (Figure 4.1).
• Record her weight and plot it on the prenatal weight gain chart (Figure 4.2).

At each subsequent visit:

- Use consistent, reliable procedures to accurately measure and record the woman's weight.
- Record her weight and plot it on the prenatal weight gain chart (Figure 4.2).
- Evaluate need to: (1) maintain current rate of weight gain; (2) increase rate of weight gain (i.e., if weight plotted is *below* normal range on weight gain chart); or (3) decrease rate of weight gain (i.e., if weight plotted is *above* normal range on weight gain chart).

Special Considerations

Inadequate weight gain is associated with low-birth-weight infants ($\leq$ 1500 gm) who demonstrate a significant increase in mortality and major morbidity (infections, ICU admissions) when compared to normal-birth-weight infants.

1. Women at risk of producing small babies—African-Americans, underweight, young adolescents—should gain weight at the *upper level* of the recommendations.
2. Women of short stature should gain weight at the *lower level* of the recommendations.
3. Twin pregnancy should be associated with a weight gain of 35–45 lbs.
4. Excessive weight gain could be a *warning sign for pre-eclampsia or hypertension and should be closely monitored.* Women who gain excessive weight without any evidence of these complications should receive professional nutritional evaluation of their intake and nutrition counseling to achieve optimal weight gain.

Charting Weight Change During Pregnancy

The Figure 4.1 chart is used to plot BMI using the patient's weight (y-axis) and height (x-axis).

The Figure 4.2 chart is used to plot patient's weight gain during each prenatal visit.

Counseling on Weight Gain During Pregnancy

1. Set a weight gain goal together with the pregnant woman, preferably at the first prenatal visit, and explain the importance of weight gain.
2. Base the recommended range of total weight gain and pattern of gain mainly on prepregnancy weight-for-height.
3. Share weight change data with the patient at each prenatal visit.

Figure 4.1
BODY MASS INDEX CHART

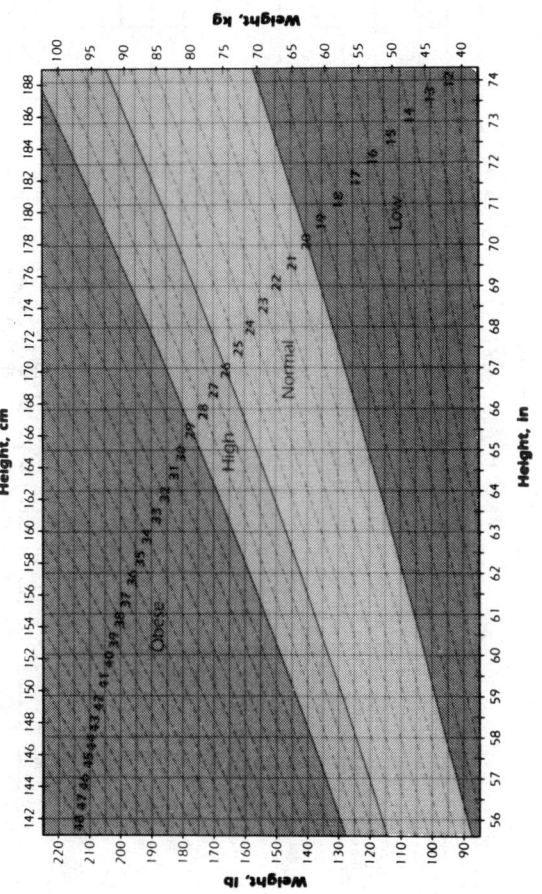

Directions

To find BMI category (e.g., obese), find the point where the woman's height and weight intersect. To estimate BMI, read the bold number on the dashed line that is closest to this point.

33

Figure 4.2
PRENATAL WEIGHT GAIN CHART

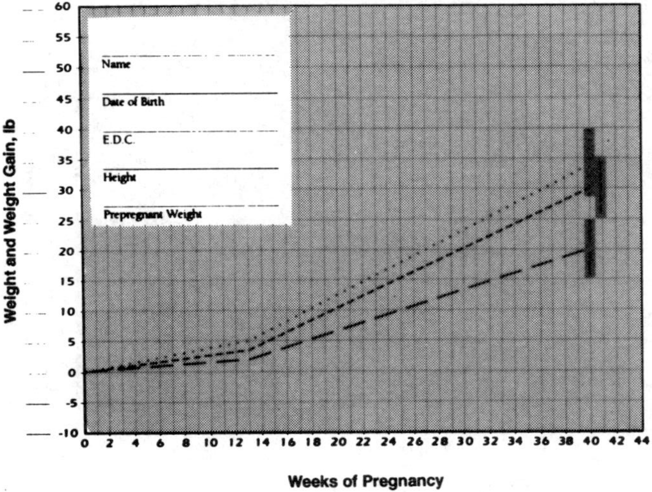

Date	Weeks of Gestation	Weight	Notes

Name
Date of Birth
E.D.C.
Height
Prepregnant Weight

Weight and Weight Gain, lb

Weeks of Pregnancy

Figures 4.1 and 4.2 reprinted with permission from Institute of Medicine. Nutrition During Pregnancy and Lactation: An Implementation Guide. Copyright 1992 by the National Academy of Sciences. Courtesy of the National Academy Press, Washington, DC.

34

Weight Changes that Signal the Need for Further Evaluation

The following weight changes have been associated with adverse outcome and therefore indicate a need for more complete medical and nutritional evaluation. Continuing patterns of less than or greater than recommended weight gain is of concern. Specifically, inadequate weight gain has been associated with low birth weight, and excessive weight gain has been associated with more difficulty with delivery and postpartum healing in women undergoing C-section deliveries.

Inadequate weight gain during pregnancy is defined as:

1. A gain of less than 2 lbs (1 kg) in any single month for women of at least moderate weight (prepregnancy BMI >19.8); or
2. A gain of less than 1 lb (0.5 kg) in any single month for obese women (prepregnancy BMI >29).

   Causes of inadequate weight gain include:
* Inadequate food supply
* Inappropriate self-restriction
* Diabetes

Excessive weight gain during pregnancy is defined as:

1. A gain of more than 6.5 lbs (3 kg) in any single month.

   Causes of excessive weight gain include:
* Multiple gestation
* Overconsumption of food
* Eclampsia
* Restricted activity

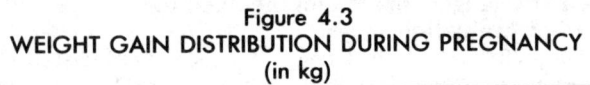

Figure 4.3
WEIGHT GAIN DISTRIBUTION DURING PREGNANCY
(in kg)

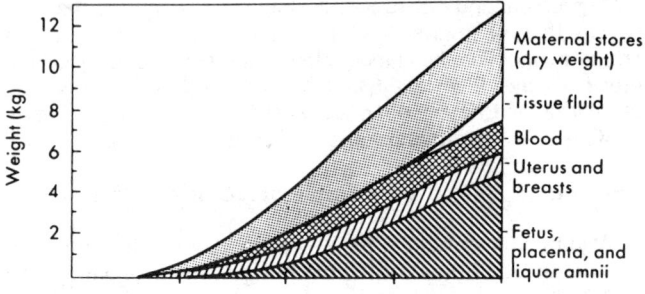

Source: Worthington-Roberts, B.S., and Williams, S.R., Nutrition in Pregnancy and Lactation, *5th ed. Mosby: St. Louis, MO, 1993, p. 74.*

Figure 4.3 and Table 4.2 provide estimates of the allocation of weight gain associated with pregnancy. It is important to realize that the data are an approximation based on limited scientific information.

Table 4.2
WEIGHT GAIN DISTRIBUTION DURING PREGNANCY
(in lbs)

Source	Pounds
Amniotic fluid	2
Baby	7–8.5
Fat/breast tissue stores for breastfeeding	1–4
Increased blood volume	4–5
Increased weight of uterus	2
Maternal fat stores	4–6
Placenta	2–2.5
Tissue fluid	3–5
TOTAL	25–35

Effects of Alcohol, Tobacco, and Illegal Drug Use on Nutritional Status and Pregnancy Outcome

Women who drink alcohol, smoke, or use illegal drugs during pregnancy place the fetus at considerable nutritional risk. The deficits induced by these substances can last a child's lifetime.

Consequences

- **Impaired growth of the fetus** (usually resulting in a weight 200–500 gm below normal full-term infants). Consumption of as few as 1–2 alcoholic beverages/day has been associated with increased incidence of low-birth-weight infants.
- **Interference with nutrient absorption, utilization, and excretion** further compromises fetal growth and nutritional status.
- **Reduced placental transport of most nutrients** is seen with alcohol consumption, smoking, or illegal drug use.
- **Increased nutrient requirements** are also seen in women who use alcohol or tobacco. Drinkers have reduced serum folate and vitamin C levels; smokers have reduced vitamin C levels.
- **Stunted growth**, which can continue into adulthood, is common. Infants born to mothers who use these substances seldom achieve their full growth potential.
- **Mental retardation or delayed development**. Infants of mothers who abuse alcohol during pregnancy are sometimes hyperactive, with short attention spans and language dysfunction.
- **Reduced fertility**. Chronic heavy drinking and smoking can interfere with fertility in both men and women and have been associated with an increased risk of spontaneous abortions.

Indications for Nutrition Referral: Pregnancy

The following is a list of referral criteria to be used in determining which obstetric patients should receive nutrition consultation.

Referral Criteria
- Anemia
- Delayed fundal height
- Excessive weight gain during pregnancy
- History of diabetes or new onset gestational diabetes Inadequate food supply or resources for food
- Inadequate weight gain
- Multiple fetus pregnancy (twins, triplets, etc.)
- Pica
- Poor dietary habits:
    a. Excess intake of fat, simple sugar, or caffeine
    b. Low intake of calcium, folate, iron, or zinc
- Pre-eclampsia
- Prepregnancy history of anorexia or bulimia
- Prepregnancy malnutrition, low weight status
- Prepregnancy obesity
- Problems with constipation, heartburn, nausea/vomiting, and so on.
- Teenage pregnancy
- Vegetarianism
- Women with nutritional questions/concerns

Table 4.3 lists risk factors for pregnancy. If the obstetric patient has a high risk indicator, she should be provided professional nutritional counseling or provided with appropriate intervention (i.e., iron supplementation for anemia).

Table 4.3
ASSESSMENT OF PRENATAL NUTRITIONAL RISK

Risk Factors for Pregnancy	Low Risk	High Risk*
Is patient economically disadvantaged or have limited income for food?	No	Yes
Is patient less than 3 years postmenarche?	No	Yes
Has patient given birth within the last year, or is she currently breastfeeding?	No	Yes
Is patient's body mass index <19.8 or >26?	No	Yes
Does patient have an unusual or nutritionally restrictive diet (vegetarian, megavitamins, pica, dieting)?	No	Yes
Is patient's calcium intake inadequate? (see Table 3.1) Four servings of milk or 4 equivalents (1 equivalent=1.5 oz cheese, 1.5 cup cottage cheese, 1cup yogurt, 1.5 cup ice cream)	No	Yes
Is patient anemic? (see Table 5.2) Hematocrit <35 mg% (1st and 2nd trimesters), <33mg% (3rd trimester)	No	Yes
Is weight gain 0.8–1.0 lb/week?	No	Yes
Is patient planning to breastfeed?	No	Yes

*All high risk indicators will require nutritional intervention/education.

Supplemental Feeding Programs
for Women, Infants, and Children

The U.S. federal government currently funds two comprehensive nutrition programs for infants, children, and pregnant women (WIC and Food Plus). These programs are administered at the county level and are summarized in Table 4.4. Referrals can be made by any health care professional. Pertinent data (hemoglobin, hematocrit, height, weight), when available, should be listed on the referral form and sent with the patient to the WIC clinic.

Table 4.4
SUMMARY OF TWO SUPPLEMENTAL FEEDING PROGRAMS*

	WIC	Food Plus
Target Audience	• Pregnant women • Breastfeeding women • Non-breastfeeding mothers of infants <6 months old • Infants <1 y/o • Children <5 y/o	• Pregnant women • Breastfeeding women • Non-breastfeeding mothers of infants <1 y/o • No infants • Children <6 y/o
Purpose	• Provide nutritious foods, health checks, referrals, nutrition education, and counseling	• Provide nutrient-rich foods and nutrition education
Eligibility Criteria	• Low income: <185% U.S. federal poverty level for women and children • County resident • Health risk (anemia, poor diet, etc.)	• Low income: <185% U.S. federal poverty level for women and children • County resident • No health risk
Food	• Nutrient rich • Limited brand names • Patient-purchased food from local supermarkets ($45/month)	• Nutrient rich • Government-purchased brand names and commodities • Warehouse distribution of 50 lbs/month
Nutrition Education	• Individual and group • Specific to risk	• Food demonstrations • Newsletters, recipes
Health Checks	• Height, weight, and anemia testing for women, infants, and children • Height, weight, and anemia testing for women and children	• None

Target audience, eligibility criteria, and services provided will vary from state to state.

41

SECTION 5
Laboratory Assessment During Pregnancy

Serum Nutrient Levels

Many laboratory values are altered during pregnancy, primarily related to hemodilution. Table 5.1 provides normal laboratory values for several tests used to assess nutritional status and/or vitamin/mineral status in pregnant and nonpregnant patients.

Table 5.1 SERUM NUTRIENT LEVELS IN PREGNANT AND NON-PREGNANT WOMEN		
Nutrient	Normal Ranges During Pregnancy	Normal Non-Pregnancy Ranges
Albumin	3.0–4.5 gm/100 ml	3.5–5.0 gm/100 ml
Calcium	4.2–5.2 mEq/dL	4.6–5.5 mEq/dL
Cholesterol	200–325 mg/100 ml	120–190 mg/100 ml
Folic acid	3–15 ng/100 ml	5–21 ng/100 ml
Glucose	<120 mg/100 ml	<110 mg/100 ml
Hemoglobin/ Hematocrit	11.1–13.5 mg/dL	12–14 mg/dL
Iron	>40 g/100 ml	>50 g/100 ml
Total iron binding capacity	300–450 g/100 ml	250–400 g/100 ml
Total protein	6.0–8.0 gm/100 ml	6.5–8.5 gm/100 ml

Adapted from Aubry, R.H., Roberts, A., and Cuenca, V. Clinical Perinatology, Vol. 2: 207, 1975.

Anemia

Anemia is a common circumstance of pregnancy. Pregnant women can demonstrate deficiency in folate, iron, and/or vitamin B_{12}. Deficiency in any one (or any combination) of these can lead to the diagnosis of anemia. Table 5.2 gives diagnostic criteria for each of the anemias and an appropriate intervention for a deficiency of any of these nutrients.

Table 5.2
DIAGNOSTIC CRITERIA AND RECOMMENDED INTERVENTIONS FOR ANEMIA

Nutrient Deficiency	Biochemical Evaluation	Dietary Assessment	Clinical Assessment	Recommended Intervention
Folate	Hgb/Hct $\Downarrow$	Diet history for intake of foods high in folate (dark green, leafy vegetables, citrus fruits).	Filiform papillary atrophy.	200–500 µg daily of unreduced pteroylglutamic acid.
	MCV, MCHC $\Uparrow$		Lobulated tongue.	Prenatal vitamins containing 400–1000 µg per tablet.
	Serum folate $\Downarrow$		Inflamed gums.	
	RBC folate $\Downarrow$			
Iron	Hgb/Hct $\Downarrow$ (normal ≥ 11 gm/dL)	Diet history for intake of foods high in iron (red meat, poultry, enriched cereals, liver).	General pallor.	Dietary counseling to improve diet.
	Serum iron $\Downarrow$	Vitamin C intake (citrus fruits, potato, tomato).	Pale mucous membranes, everted eyelids.	30–60 mg iron daily with food.
	Total iron binding $\Uparrow$	Excessive consumption of tea or coffee.	Spoon nails.	
	Serum ferritin $\Downarrow$	High intake of bran.		

Table 5.2
DIAGNOSTIC CRITERIA AND RECOMMENDED INTERVENTIONS FOR ANEMIA *Continued*

Nutrient Deficiency	Biochemical Evaluation	Dietary Assessment	Clinical Assessment	Recommended Intervention
Vitamin B₁₂	Hgb/Hct ⇓ MCV, MCHC ⇑ Serum B₁₂ ⇓	Diet history for intake of foods high in vitamin B₁₂ (meats, milk, cheese, eggs).	Weakness, fatigue, red swollen tongue, paresthesia, anorexia, loss of taste.	Dietary lack: 1–3 µg B₁₂ taken orally each day. Malabsorption: 150–300 µg B₁₂ by injection each month.
Combined Deficiency	Hgb/Hct ⇓ or normal MCV, MCHC ⇑, ⇓, or within normal limits Serum B₁₂ ⇓ Serum ferritin ⇓	Diet history for generalized inadequate diet, alcohol consumption, malabsorption syndromes.	See above.	See above. Supplement with nutrients as indicated.

SECTION 6
Nutrition-Related Concerns

Common Complaints During Pregnancy

Many pregnant women experience minor problems during pregnancy which may impact upon their eating. Listed below are several of the more common concerns and appropriate interventions to relieve symptoms.

Constipation
- Drink plenty of fluids.
- Increase fiber intake (see Table 3.2).
- Increase activity as tolerated.
- Use of Colace® or Metamucil® may be used—under the advice of the physician—if dietary changes are not effective.
- Supplement with additional iron only when indicated.

Heartburn
- Eat small, frequent meals.
- Eat slowly and chew food thoroughly.
- Avoid highly seasoned, spicy foods.
- Wear loose-fitting clothing that does not bind at waist.
- Remain seated during meals and 30 minutes after.
- Avoid caffeine (see Table 6.1).
- Reduce intake of high-fat foods or added fat.
- Avoid gas-forming foods and chewing gum.

Lactose Intolerance
- Try smaller amounts of lactose-containing foods at a time.
- Eat lower lactose foods such as cheese, cottage cheese, and yogurt.
- Try lactase enzyme replacements such as Lact-Aid® and Dairy Ease®.

Nausea
- Avoid fried or gas-forming foods.
- Avoid large meals; eat small, frequent meals.
- Eat crackers or dry cereal before rising from bed in the morning.
- Drink fluids between meals, not with meals.
- Avoid highly seasoned, spicy foods.
- Avoid strong cooking odors such as fish, sauerkraut, etc.
- Take vitamins/minerals *with* food.
- Sip on mineral or soda water.
- Eat slowly.

Weight Gain, Inadequate
- Eat more frequently.
- Choose nutrient dense foods such as meats, dairy products, peanut butter, breads and cereals, etc.
- Add margarine, butter, sauces, sour cream, cream cheese, gravy, etc., to foods for additional calories.
- Use liquid nutritional supplements if necessary.
- Keep records of food intake for evaluation by the dietitian.
- Avoid alcohol, tobacco use.
- Avoid caffeine.
- Limit activity.

Weight Gain, Excessive
- Limit intake of sweets.
- Limit intake of foods high in fat.
- Avoid adding margarine, butter, sauces, sour cream, or gravy to food.
- Use low-fat or fat-free food items.
- Increase activity as tolerated.
- Reduce portion sizes.
- Keep records of food intake for evaluation by the dietitian.
- Chart weight gain on a weight gain curve chart (see Figure 4.2).
- Select healthy snacks such as fresh fruits and vegetables, low-fat crackers or cookies, and low-fat dairy products.
- Avoid sugar-containing beverages (colas, Kool-Aid®, fruit drinks, etc.).

Exercise During Pregnancy

Exercising during pregnancy can promote good muscle tone, cardiovascular strength, and reduce fatigue. Regular exercise throughout pregnancy can also make the delivery easier by increasing stamina. Following are recommendations for women who exercise during pregnancy.

Recommendations*
- Physician and patient should discuss exercise early in the pregnancy.
- Exercise regularly—at least three times each week is preferable to intermittent exercise.
- Stop exercising when fatigued and not exercise to exhaustion.
- Preexercise warm-up and postexercise cool-downs are important.
- No exercise should be completed in the supine position after the first trimester.
- Wear comfortable shoes.
- Wear clothing which does not restrict activity.
- Caloric intake should be adequate to meet additional caloric requirements of the pregnancy *and* the exercise.
- Maintain hydration/drink small amounts frequently throughout exercise.
- Walking, swimming and stationery bicycles will minimize risk of injury.
- Avoid starting a new sport which is strenuous increases the potential for even mild abdominal trauma and/or which the mother did not participate in prior to pregnancy.

*Adapted from *American College of Obstetricians and Gynecologists,* Guidelines for Exercise in Pregnancy and Postpartum Period.

Caffeine

Effects of Caffeine During Pregnancy

Across several studies, there is no clear evidence that caffeine is related to problems during pregnancy or birth defects. However, caffeine is not an essential nutrient and, therefore, there is no reason to recommend caffeine intake. There is a small amount of evidence that heavy caffeine consumption may reduce zinc and iron absorption, increase urinary calcium excretion, and reduce total caloric intake. In addition, it is important to be aware that caffeine is transferred through the placenta to the fetus where it remains for a significantly longer time span than in the maternal body. The generally accepted recommendation from health professionals for caffeine intake is <300 mg/day or <3 cups/day (see Table 6.1).

Table 6.1 CAFFEINE CONTENT OF SELECTED FOODS/BEVERAGES		
Food/Beverage Item	Serving Size	Caffeine Content (mg)
Cafe Amaretto	6 oz	60
Chocolate cake	1/16th of 9-in. cake	14
Cocoa	8 oz (= 1 cup)	13–24
Coffee:		
Decaffeinated	8 oz	3–7
Ground/Brewed	8 oz	100–250
Instant	8 oz	65–95
Cola	12 oz	30–65
Jolt Cola®	12 oz	90
KitKat® candy bar	1.5 oz bar	5
Mountain Dew®	12 oz	54
Tea	8 oz	35–85

Effects of Caffeine During Lactation

The level of caffeine in breast milk is 1.5-3% of the amount the mother ingests. If a mother drinks more than 6-8 cups of coffee per day, her baby can accumulate enough caffeine to display symptoms such as irritability and sleeplessness.

Sugar Substitutes

The use of sugar substitutes during pregnancy remains controversial. Several scientific studies have failed to show any adverse effects of aspartame (Equal®) during pregnancy on either the mother or the fetus. Most clinicians recommend a daily intake of ≤2 servings of foods or beverages containing aspartame. Because of the high phenylalanine content, pregnant women with PKU should only consume aspartame if the intake level is within their daily allowance for phenylalanine.

Saccharin (Sugar Twin®, Sweet One®, Sweet-n-Low®) has been shown to cause cancer in laboratory animals; therefore, most clinicians recommend avoiding foods or beverages containing saccharine during pregnancy. Use of sunette (Ascesulfame-K®) has also failed to show any adverse effects. Because it is also controversial and not a necessary nutrient, exposure should be limited to ≤2 servings/day.

SECTION 7
Gestational
Diabetes Mellitus

Gestational Diabetes Mellitus

Gestational Diabetes Mellitus (GDM) is carbohydrate intolerance of variable severity with onset or first recognition during pregnancy. GDM is usually identified in mid- to late-pregnancy and seems to relate to increased levels of anti-insulinemic hormones—specifically estrogen, prolactin, progesterone, cortisol, and human placenta lactogen. If GDM is not controlled, there is increased risk for large babies, and labor or postpartum complications. GDM generally poses little threat for congenital anomalies.

The first line of treatment for GDM is usually dietary changes. If fasting glucose levels are unusually elevated, insulin may be started immediately. With or without insulin therapy, diet therapy will be essential to the total care of the patient.

Screening Criteria*
1. Glucose measurement in plasma.
2. 50 gm oral glucose load—administered between the 24th and 28th weeks of pregnancy and without regard to time of day or time of last meal—to all pregnant women who have not been identified as having glucose intolerance before the 24th week.
3. Venous plasma glucose measured one hour later.
4. A value of ≥140 mg/dL in venous plasma indicates the need for a full diagnostic glucose tolerance test.

Diagnostic Criteria*
1. 100 gm oral glucose load—administered in the morning after overnight fast for at least 8 hours but not more than 14 hours, and after at least 3 days of unrestricted diet (≥150gm carbohydrate) and physical activity.
2. Venous plasma glucose measured fasting and at 1-, 2-, and 3-hours post-glucose load administration. Subject should remain seated and not smoke throughout the test.

Reprinted with permission from Diabetes , Vol. 34, Suppl. 2, 1985. Copyright © 1985 by American Diabetes Association, Inc.

3. Two or more of the following venous plasma glucose concentrations must be met or exceeded for positive diagnosis:
   Fasting, 105 mg/dL
   1-hour post-glucose load, 190 mg/dL
   2-hours post-glucose load, 165 mg/dL
   3-hours post-glucose load, 145 mg/dL

Treatment

Diet Therapy

Table 7.1 SAMPLE MENU* FOR THE PATIENT WITH GDM		
Breakfast	*Lunch*	*Dinner*
1 starch/bread	2 starch/bread	2 starch
1 meat, medium fat	2 meat	3 meat
1 fat	1 vegetable	2 vegetable
1 milk, non-fat	1 fruit	1 milk
	1 milk, non-fat	2 fat
	1 fat	
Breakfast	*Afternoon Snack*	*Evening Snack*
1 fruit	1 starch	1 starch/bread
1 starch/bread	1 fat	1 milk, non-fat
1 fat		1 fat

Daily intake of 2000 calories: 47% carbohydrates; 22% protein; 31% fat.

Insulin Therapy

Table 7.2
INSULIN ADJUSTMENT IN GDM: HYPERGLYCEMIA

Time/Blood glucose		Insulin Adjustments
Prebreakfast	**Bed NPH**	**Breakfast Regular**
BS <70	⟱ NPH by 2 units	⟱ Breakfast Regular by 2 units
71–100	No change in NPH	No change in calculated Breakfast Regular
101–140	⟰ NPH by 2 units	⟰ Breakfast Regular by 2 units
>140	⟰ NPH by 4 units	⟰ Breakfast Regular by 4 units
1 Hour After Breakfast		
BS >141		⟰ Breakfast Regular for the following day by 2 units
1 Hour After lunch	**Breakfast NPH**	
BS >141	⟰ Breakfast NPH by 2units or ⟱ Lunch carbohydrate	
Predinner	**Breakfast NPH**	**Dinner Regular**
BS <70	⟱ NPH by 2 units	⟱ Dinner Regular by 2 units
71–100	No change in NPH	No change in calculated Dinner Regular
101–140	⟰ NPH by 2 units	⟰ Dinner regular by 2 units
>141	⟰ NPH by 4 units	⟰ Dinner regular by 4 units
1 Hour After Dinner		
BS >141		⟰ Dinner Regular for the following day by 2 units

Tables 7.1 and 7.2 adapted from Jovanovic-Peterson, L., and Peterson, C.M. *When to Start Insulin in the Gestational Diabetic.* Diabetes Professional, Summer 1988, p.8–9.

SECTION 8
Postpartum
Nutritional Care

Postpartum and Lactation

Postpartum is a time full of adjustments and concerns for the new mother. Nutritional care of the new mother during this time should focus on:
• Healing.
• Promoting and enhancing the breastfeeding experience.
• Reassuring patient's diet efforts to "get back in shape."

Health care professionals play a primary role in a mother's decision to breastfeed. Research has shown that, in particular, first-time mothers frequently look to their physician or other health care professionals for guidance on not only whether or not to breastfeed but also on how to breastfeed. The next several pages provide information to support the new mother in her decision to breastfeed her infant.

Advantages of Breastfeeding
• Breast milk is nutritionally superior to any alternative.
• Breast milk contains immunoglobulins and maternal antibodies, including macrophages, lymphocytes, B-cells, T-cells, IgA, IgG, and IgM.
• Breast milk is bacteriologically safe and always fresh.
• Breast milk is the least allergenic of any infant food.
• Breastfed infants have lower rates of diarrhea and other infections, including otitis media.
• Breast milk promotes G.I. tract maturation.
• Breastfeeding promotes jaw and tooth development.
• Breastfed babies are less likely to be overfed.
• Breast milk is less expensive.
• Breastfeeding promotes infant-maternal bonding.
• Although postpartum weight loss occurs at a similar rate, breastfeeding women lose proportionally more lower body fat mass than do non-breastfeeding women.

Obstacles of Lactating
• Lack of support from family members—spouse, mother, sibling, etc.
• Lack of postpartum professional support to breastfeed
• Inadequate education on breastfeeding
• Breast regarded only in its sexual context, at the exclusion of its physiological role.
• Pacifiers.
• Preoccupation with dietary intake (i.e., feel they should not breastfeed because their dietary habits are not perfectly matched to Food Guide Pyramid).

Postpartum Healing

In order to promote adequate healing, particularly in mothers who have had a C-section, the postpartum mother should be encouraged to eat a well-balanced diet. Adequate intakes of protein, zinc, vitamin A, and vitamin C are essential to the healing process; thus food items rich in these nutrients should be liberally included in the postpartum daily diet (see tables in Section3). Many physicians also recommend continuing multivitamin/mineral supplements, once daily, for up to 6 weeks postpartum.

Postpartum Weight Loss

Most mother are anxious to lose weight and get back into shape after child birth. It is important that new mothers adhere to the following recommendations:
- Remember, it took 9 months to gain the additional weight. A realistic goal for getting back into shape is 9 months.
- Keep weight loss expectations at a reasonable level (>4.5 lbs/month is *not* reasonable or advisable).
- Avoid quick weight loss diets which may delay healing or dehydrate the mother. This is crucial particularly to the breastfeeding mother and especially during the first 3-5 weeks of lactation.
- Include daily exercise in any weight loss regime.
- Continue taking a daily multivitamin/mineral supplement to supply 100% RDA.
- If breastfeeding, maintain caloric intake >1600 kcal/day to assure adequate milk supply.
- Select low-fat alternatives when purchasing food items.
- Increased fiber intake—such as fresh fruits, raw vegetables, whole grains and whole grain breads and cereals, and low-fat dairy products—will not only enhance nutritional intake but will also help curb appetite and promote weight loss.
- Decrease intake of high-fat foods (margarine, sauces, gravies, fatty meats, whole milk, fried foods, pastries/doughnuts, cakes/pies, and many fast foods).
- Drink plenty of calorie-free, caffeine-free beverages such as herbal teas, water, decaffeinated coffee, etc.
- Breastfeeding women lose weight at the same rate as women who do not breastfeed; however, breastfeeding women tend

to lose more lower body fat mass (another benefit of breastfeeding).

Table 8.1 will be useful in recommending healthy snacks for the postpartum woman.

Table 8.1 NUTRITIOUS SNACKS OF 100 CALORIES OR LESS	
Food Item	*Serving Size*
Bagel	1/2
Carrot, raw	1 cup or 1 large
Cheese, low-fat	1 oz
Cottage cheese, low-fat	1/3 cup
Entenmann's® fat-free cakes/pastries	1 small slice
Figs, low-fat or other Newton® cookies	1-1/2
Fruit, dried (like apricots, raisins, prunes)	4 Tbsp
Fruit, fresh	1 medium
Graham crackers	2
Milk, skim	1 cup
Pretzels	15
Pudding made w/skim milk	1/3 cup
Rice cakes, flavored	2
Tortilla chips, baked, low-fat and w/salsa	12
Yogurt, frozen	1/2 cup
Yogurt, low-fat	1/2 cup

Postpartum Exercise

Exercise is a key component of postpartum care. Many women will *want* to begin an exercise program to enhance fitness, whereas others will need encouragement. Listed below are guidelines for including exercise in postpartum care:

- Regular exercise at least three times/week is preferable.
- A well-fitting support bra should be worn during exercises.
- Liquids should be taken liberally before and after exercise to prevent dehydration. If necessary, activity should be interrupted to replenish fluids.
- Heart rate should be measured at times of peak activity.
- Activity should be stopped and the physician consulted if any unusual symptoms appear.
- For the woman who has had a C-section, abdominal exercises should be avoided during the first 6 weeks postpartum.
- Women who have sedentary life-styles should begin with physical activity at very low intensity and advance activity levels very gradually.
- Jerky, bouncy movements should be avoided.
- Deep flexion or extension of joints should be avoided because of connective tissue laxity.
- Care should be taken to gradually rise from floor to avoid orthostatic hypotension.
- Vigorous exercise should be preceded by 5 minutes of muscle warm-up.
- Vigorous exercise should be followed by a period of gradually declining activity that includes stationary stretching.
- Vigorous exercise should not be performed in hot, humid weather or during periods of febrile illness.

Diet During Lactation

Caloric Requirements

Lactating women need an additional 500 kcal/day on average to produce the quantity of breast milk needed for normal infant growth and development. (If pregnancy weight gain was inadequate, additional caloric intake of 650 kcal/day is recommended during lactation.) In order to meet the additional micronutrient needs of lactation, the mother will need to select nutrient-rich food items (see tables in Section 3). In addition, the mother should be encouraged to select foods which are not high in fat, thus not supplying excessive calories.

Extra nutrients are best obtained in the form of between-meal snacks such as: half a sandwich and a glass of low-fat milk; cottage cheese with fresh fruit and juice; or low-fat yogurt, fresh fruit, and low-fat milk.

Protein Requirements

Lactating mothers need an additional 15 gm of protein daily. This should come from low-fat food items so as not to promote excessive caloric intake. Most women eat plenty of protein even without making a conscientious effort to do so.

Some examples of low-fat food items are low-fat dairy products such as skim milk, low-fat cottage cheese, low-fat yogurt, low-fat cheese; lean meats such as fish, lean beef, white meat chicken or turkey; and a variety of vegetable protein sources.

General Recommendations

- Drink plenty of fluids—drink to thirst. Excessive fluid intake will not increase milk supply, but inadequate intake *will* restrict it.
- Drink three servings of milk daily.
- Eat a variety of foods daily—fruits, vegetables, breads/cereals/grains, dairy products, and meats.
- Avoid rapid weight loss (>4.5 lbs/month is *not* advised).
- Try to consume at least one source of vitamin A daily—cantaloupe, carrots, spinach, sweet potatoes, mangoes, or pumpkin (see Table 3.8).
- Avoid caffeine.
- Remember: Don't be too concerned about consuming the "perfect" diet. Too much anxiety about diet may actually decrease milk production.
- Adequate breast milk can be produced despite adverse circumstances.

Foods/Beverages Consumed During Lactation Which May Cause Infant G.I. Distress

All foods are acceptable to eat during lactation, but occasionally an infant will be bothered by something the mother has eaten. Table 8.2 contains a list of some foods and beverages that may possibly be problematic. If an infant has frequent colic, the mother should be advised to avoid the listed foods on a trial basis in order to determine if a change in diet reduces infant colic. If whole food groups are omitted, the mother should see a dietitian to assure adequate nutrition.

Table 8.2
FOODS AND BEVERAGES WHICH MAY CAUSE G.I. DISTRESS TO BREASTFEEDING INFANTS

Consumed in any amount:	*Consumed in large amounts:*
Chocolate	Beans
Coffee	Broccoli
Colas	Cabbage
Tea	Cauliflower
Other caffeine sources	Garlic
	Onion
Consumed in large amounts, these may also cause indigestion or diarrhea:	*If family history of allergies:*
Fresh fruits	Milk
Fresh juices	Wheat

Indications for Nutrition
Referral: Lactation

- Patient-expressed concerns related to breastfeeding.
- Predelivery or immediate postpartum breastfeeding counseling.
- Postpartum weight gain.
- Excessive weight loss during lactation (i.e., >4.5 lbs/month).
- Mother's weight falling below normal weight-for-height or prepregnancy weight.
- Slow infant growth.
- Restrictive food practices possibly to prevent infant colic, allergies, excessive weight gain.
- Inadequate access to food.
- Excessive caffeine intake.
- Inadequate fluid intake.
- Anemia.
- Evidence of excessive vitamin/mineral supplementation.
- Multiple births (twins, triplets).

Breastfeeding Basics Algorithm

The success of breastfeeding depends on the infant's ability to stimulate the breast, ingest, digest, and metabolize the milk, and the mother's ability to produce and provide adequate access to the milk. One of the most important facts to know about breastfeeding is that it works on a *law of supply and demand*. Frequent and unrestricted access to the breast will determine the amount of breast milk produced. Intervention, such as formula supplementation, will interfere with the infant's desire or ability to nurse. This will reduce milk production. The breastfeeding thriving chart (Figure 8.1) details the components of successful breastfeeding.

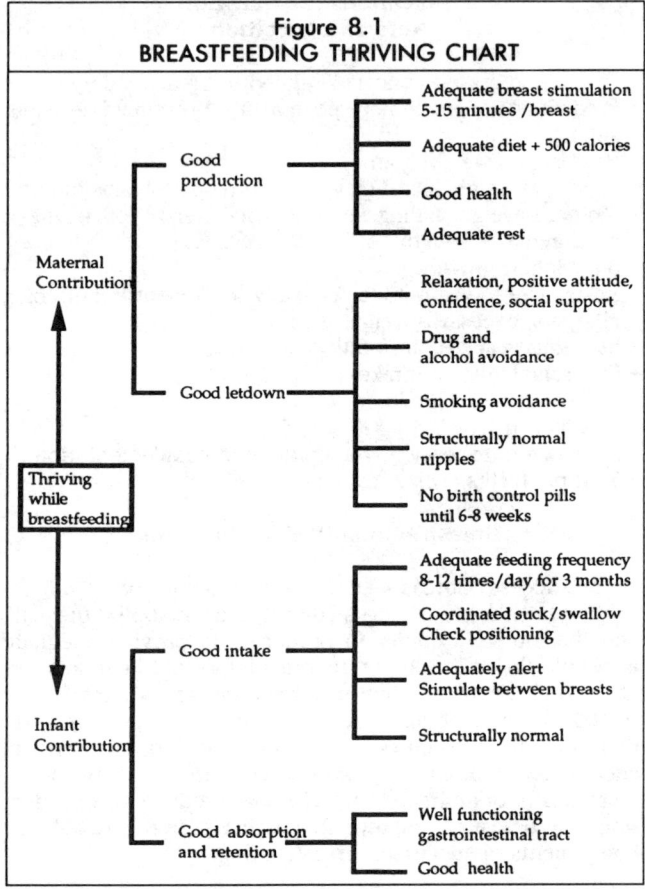

Figure 8.1
BREASTFEEDING THRIVING CHART

How to Respond to Breastfeeding Concerns

Breastfeeding mothers may need your help in addressing their concerns related to breastfeeding. Table 8.3 offers some breastfeeding tips which are appropriate to use with your patients.

Breastfeeding Resources

For more information on breastfeeding, you can contact:
- Local child birth education associations
- County health department
- Local hospitals
- Nutrition services or lactation specialists
- La Leche League 708-455-7730
- Medela Breastfeeding Products 1-800-435-8316

Table 8.3
BREASTFEEDING TIPS

Concern	Recommended Action
Breast Care	Nipple pulling, tugging, or rolling during pregnancy is not necessary to prepare for breastfeeding. Avoid soaps or lotions to the nipples. Air dry nipples after breastfeeding.
Breast Creams	Vitamin E, breast creams, or ointments are not recommended. They have not been shown to heal the nipple and can make soreness worse by keeping the nipple moist (see "Nipples, Sore").
Breast Surgery	Any type of breast surgery may interfere with milk supply. Consult with a lactation consultant and/or your doctor for individual advice.
Cesarean Section	Breastfeed your baby as soon as possible after delivery, preferably in the recovery room. Hold your baby in a comfortable position. Use pillows across your abdomen to protect the incision and support your baby. You will need additional rest at home.
Duration of Breastfeeding: How long and how often?	Breastfeed every 2–3 hours for at least 10–15 minutes on each breast. Watch your baby for signs that he is full, like falling asleep, losing interest in feeding, or stopping breastfeeding. Your breast is never completely empty. It is alright to switch breasts several times during a feeding.

Table 8.3
BREASTFEEDING TIPS   Continued

Concern	Recommended Action
Engorgement	Engorgement may occur when milk first comes in or when feedings are missed or delayed. Use warm compresses or shower before feedings. Hand express to soften areola, making it easier for your baby to latch on. Breastfeed every 1–2 hours for 10–20 minutes per breast. Apply ice to breast and under arm after feeding until swelling decreases. Take non-aspirin pain reliever. If no relief in 48 hours, call lactation consultant or doctor.
Early First Feeding	Put baby to your breast soon after delivery, if possible within the first 2 hours. Cuddling, licking, and brief sucking are good signs that you and your baby are learning to breastfeed. Offer your breast often to let your baby practice. Ask a supportive nurse for help.
Extra Feedings	Healthy breastfed newborns do not need formula, water, or juice. Breastfeed at least every 2–3 hours during the first month. Older breastfed babies will be ready for solid foods and juices between 4–6 months of age.
Hospital Survival Skills	"Rooming-in" with your baby is your right as a consumer. Keep your baby with you as much as possible so you can breastfeed often. Do not give bottles. Do not limit feeding time at your breast. Ask a supportive nurse for help. Do not accept formula gift packs.

continued on next page

Table 8.3
BREASTFEEDING TIPS *Continued*

Concern	Recommended Action
Is Baby Getting Enough Milk?	Your body makes as much milk as your baby needs. Signs that a newborn is getting enough breast milk are 6–8 wet diapers a day, baby sleeps some between feedings, and baby gains 3–7 oz/week. Babies less than 4 weeks old should have at least one bowel movement a day. Older babies may go 3–4 days between bowel movements.
Jaundice	Try to breastfeed at least every 2 hours around the clock. If breastfeeding is stopped, pump your breasts to maintain milk supply. Avoid water or formula feedings. Consult your baby's doctor.
Latch-on	Latch-on is necessary for baby to begin sucking at your breast. Poor latch-on is a major cause of sore nipples. Baby's mouth should be at nipple level. Support your breast by placing the thumb on the top and four fingers underneath. Tickle baby's bottom lip with nipple until baby opens mouth very wide. Center your nipple quickly and bring baby very close to you. Baby's nose and chin should be touching your breast.
Leaking	Leaking is a sign of normal letdown in the early weeks of breastfeeding. You may use breast pads in your bra between feedings. Avoid pads with plastic lining. During sexual activity, leaking may occur; you may wish to breastfeed your baby first.

Table 8.3 *Continued*

BREASTFEEDING TIPS *Continued*

Concern	Recommended Action
Mastitis	Mastitis is a swollen, inflamed, or infected area in the breast. Watch for flu-like symptoms such as fever above 101°F, chills and muscle aches, and a reddened, hot, tender or swollen area in the breast. Rest, breastfeed often, and drink more fluids. Contact your doctor, as antibiotics may be needed. **Do not stop breastfeeding.**
Myths and Misconception	The truth is: Breast sagging is not a result of breastfeeding. Breast size does not affect ability to breastfeed. Drinking beer, Manzanilla tea, or large amounts of fluids does not make more milk.
Nipples, Flat or Inverted (before birth)	Flat or inverted nipples retract or move in toward the breast. Breast shells (milk cups) may be worn during pregnancy to help minimize inverted nipples. Gradually increase time of use from a few hours to 8–10 hours/day. Do not wear while sleeping. Air dry nipples if leaking occurs. Breast shells should not be used by women at risk for preterm labor. Check with your doctor.
Nipples, Flat or Inverted (after birth)	Begin breastfeeding as soon as possible after birth. Breastfeed frequently to avoid engorgement. Use nipple rolling or stretching before each breastfeeding. Pump your breast for a short period before breastfeeding, or try ice wrapped in a cloth and placed on the nipple before feeding. Breast shells (milk cups) may be used between feedings. Remove the breast shell just before placing baby at your breast.

continued on next page

Table 8.3
BREASTFEEDING TIPS *Continued*

Concern	Recommended Action
Nipples, Rubber	Avoid rubber nipples for the first several weeks of breastfeeding. Babies may be confused by the rubber nipple and refuse to breastfeed. Pacifiers should not be used as a substitute for frequent breastfeeding.
Nipple Shields	Nipple shields are soft plastic or rubber devices designed to be placed over the human nipple. Nipple shields interfere with milk production and may result in poor weight gain in your baby. They may confuse baby on how to breastfeed. Nipple shields are not recommended (see "Rubber Nipples").
Nipples, Sore	Nipple tenderness commonly occurs, but breastfeeding should not be painful. Correct latch-on and proper positioning can prevent or minimize soreness. If nipples are sore: vary baby's position on your breast; air dry nipples after feeding; avoid soap, alcohol, or nipple creams; use shorter, more frequent feedings; use the least sore breast first; rub a few drops of breast milk on the nipple after feeding.
Plugged Duct	A plugged duct is a tender or sore lump in the breast. Common causes: tight bra; sleeping on stomach; poor positioning; delayed/infrequent breastfeeding. Feed every 2–3 hours. Apply warm, moist heat 10–15 minutes before feeding. Massage your breast before and during feeding. Change baby's position each feeding. Take non-aspirin pain reliever. Untreated plugged ducts may lead to mastitis.

Table 8.3
BREASTFEEDING TIPS   *Continued*

Concern	Recommended Action
Position of Mother	Relax in a comfortable position with extra pillows for support. Do not lean over baby; bring baby to your breast.
Position of Baby—Cradle Hold	Hold your baby with his/her head resting in the bend of your arm. Baby's face, chest, shoulder, and knees should all be facing youyou should be tummy to tummy. Your arm should support your baby's bottom or upper thigh. Baby needs to remain at breast level.
Position of Baby—Football Hold	Support baby by your side with one or two pillows. Baby's bottom should touch the chair or bed; his/her legs should extend upward. Your arm will support baby's back, and your hand should firmly support the base of your baby's head. Baby's mouth should be at nipple level.

Adapted from Nutrition Council of Arizona Breastfeeding Advocates. Breastfeeding Helper. *Copyright © 1991.*

References and Suggested Readings

Albert, M.B., and Callaway, C.W. *Clinical Nutrition for the House Officer*. Williams & Wilkins: Baltimore, MD, 1992.

American College of Obstetricians and Gynecologists. Exercise during pregnancy and the postpartum period. ACOG Technical Bulletin 189. Washington DC: ACOG, 1994.

Arizona Department of Health Services, Office of Nutrition Services. *Nutrition and Pregnancy Guidelines*, 1990.

Arizona Dietetic Association, Inc. *Arizona Diet Manual*, Arizona Dietetic Association, Inc., Phoenix, AZ, 1992.

Aubry, R.H., Roberts, A., and Cuenca, V. *Clinical Perinatology* 2:207, 1975.

Dimperio, D. *Prenatal Nutrition: Clinical Guidelines for Nurses*. March of Dimes Birth Defect Foundation: White Plains, NY, 1988.

Freinkel, N. (Ed.). Proceedings of the Second International Workshop Conference on Gestational Diabetes Mellitus, American Diabetes Association Inc. *Diabetes* 34(Suppl 2): 123–126, 1985.

Henry, A.K., and Feldhausen, J. *Drugs, Vitamins & Minerals in Pregnancy*. Fisher Books: Tucson, AZ, 1989.

Huggins, K. *The Nursing Mother's Companion*. The Harvard Common Press, Cambridge, MA, 1986.

Institute of Medicine, Subcommittee for a Clinical Application Guide. *Nutrition During Pregnancy and Lactation: An Implementation Guide*. National Academy Press: Washington, DC, 1992.

Institute of Medicine, Subcommittee on Nutritional Status and Weight Gain During Pregnancy. *Nutrition During Pregnancy*. National Academy Press: Washington, DC, 1990.

Institute of Medicine, Subcommittee on Nutrition During Lactation. *Nutrition During Lactation*. National Academy Press: Washington, DC, 1991.

Jovanovic-Peterson, L., and Peterson, C.M. Dietary Manipulation as a Primary Strategy for Pregnancies Complicated by Diabetes. *J Am Coll Nutr* 9:320–325, 1990.

Jovanovic-Peterson, L., and Peterson, C.M. When to Start Insulin in the Gestational Diabetic. *Diabetes Professional* 8–9, Summer 1988.

Kalkhoff, R.K. Impact of Maternal Fuels and Nutritional State on Fetal Growth. *Diabetes* 40:561-565, 1991.

Katch, F.I., and McArdle, W.D. *Introduction to Nutrition, Exercise, and Health*, 4th ed. Lea & Febiger: Philadelphia, 1993.

La Leche League International. *The Breastfeeding Answer Book*. La Leche League International, Franklin Park, IL, 1992.

Lagua, R., and Claudio, V. *Nutiriton and Diet Therapy Handbook*, 4e, Chapman & Hall: New York, 1996.

Laurence, R. *Breastfeeding: A Guide for the Medical Profession*. Mosby: St. Louis, MO, 1989.

Mason, D., and Ingersoll, D. *Breastfeeding and the Working Mother*. St. Martins Press, New York, 1986.

National Academy of Sciences-National Research Council. *Recommended Dietary Allowances*, 10th ed. National Academy Press: Washington, DC, 1990.

Nutrition Council of Arizona Breastfeeding Advocates. *Breastfeeding Helper*, Nutrition Council of Arizona Breastfeeding Advocates, Tucson, AZ, 1991 [Pamphlet].

Pennington, J.A.T. *Bowes and Church's Food Values of Portions Commonly Used*, 16th ed. J.B. Lippincott: Philadelphia, 1994.

U.S. Department of Agriculture and the U.S. Department of Health and Human Services. *Food Guide Pyramid: A Guide to Daily Food Choices*. National Live Stock and Meat Board, Washington, DC, 1993.

Weinsier, R.L., and Morgan, S.L. *Fundamentals of Clinical Nutrition*. Mosby: St. Louis, MO, 1993.

Worthington-Roberts, B.S., and Williams, S.R. *Nutrition in Pregnancy and Lactation*, 5th ed. Mosby: St. Louis, MO, 1993.

Index